The Sesamoiditis Cure

A definitive guide to understanding and
overcoming ball of foot pain.

By Greg Unger

2ND EDITION

Contact Information:

Website: www.thesesamoiditiscure.com

Contact Email: businessathlete101@gmail.com

Ordering Information:

Quantity sales. Special discounts are available on quantity purchases by corporations, associations, and others. For details, please email businessathlete101@gmail.com or visit www.thesesamoiditiscure.com.

Dedication

Thank you to all of the medical professional, friends and family who helped me write this book. I spent quite some time compiling the best information I could find as well as being the best guinea pig I could be in order to present the best information possible.

I'd especially like to thank my sister who did a brilliant job fixing my original mess. My father also spent quite a bit of time making necessary corrections. Let's just say it was a family effort.

TABLE OF CONTENTS

CHAPTER 1   LET ME START OUT BY SAYING 1

CHAPTER 2   AN ATTITUDE ADJUSTMENT 5

CHAPTER 3   WHAT ARE SESAMOIDS? 7

CHAPTER 4   TYPES OF SESAMOID INJURIES IN THE FOOT 9

CHAPTER 5   WHAT IS SESAMOIDITIS? 11

WHAT IS A BONE SCAN? 13

CHAPTER 6   CAUSES OF SESAMOIDITIS 14

CHAPTER 7   SYMPTOMS OF SESAMOIDITIS 16

CHAPTER 8   THE DIAGNOSIS OF SESAMOIDITIS 17

CHAPTER 9   THE "USUAL" TREATMENT OF SESAMOIDITIS 19

TREATMENT PROTOCOL FOR SESAMOIDITIS 19

CONSERVATIVE TREATMENT TECHNIQUES INCLUDE: 20

CHAPTER 10   SESAMOID FRACTURE, A SLIGHTLY DIFFERENT BEAST 22

TREATMENT FOR A SESAMOID FRACTURE 24

CHAPTER 11   THE FIRST THING YOU NEED TO DO 25

CHAPTER 12   A SUMMARY OF WHAT WE'RE DEALING WITH 27

CHAPTER 13   STEP BY STEP GUIDE TO BEATING SESAMOIDITIS 28

FOR NON-FRACTURE SESAMOIDITIS 28

     Step 1 - Stop causing pain and inflammation to your forefoot. 28

     Step 2 – Know what you are dealing with. 29

     Step 3 - Stop additional damage 31

     Step 4 - Get rid of inflammation 31

     Step 5 – Make sure the problem is gone before you do things normally 31

THE FOLLOWING TREATMENT PLAN SHOULD BE FOLLOWED IMMEDIATELY. 32

     Preparation 32

The Plan 33

CHAPTER 14   THE ROLE OF NUTRITION AND CALCIUM..**36**

THE INGREDIENTS THAT CAN HELP 40

CHAPTER 15   A COMPREHENSIVE LIST OF MODALITIES **43**

CALCIUM 44

ACUPUNCTURE 46

ACUPUNCTURE WITH E-STIM.. 48

ICING, BAG OF ICE, STRAPS, DIXIE CUP 49

FOOT ICE BATHS USING A STORAGE CONTAINER 50

TAPING THE BIG TOE DOWN 52

SHOELACES 53

DAS BOOT! (THE BOOT!).. 54

DANCER PADS 55

SESAMOID WRAP.. 56

METATARSAL PADS... 57

FELT PADDING 58

TENS DEVICE 59

ULTRASOUND 61

COLD LASER THERAPY 62

SHOCKWAVE THERAPY.. 63

EXTRACORPOREAL SHOCK WAVE THERAPY (ESWT) 65

OVER THE COUNTER ORTHOTICS 67

CUSTOM ORTHOTICS FROM A SPORTS PODIATRIST.. 68

CUSTOM ORTHOTICS FROM A PEDORTHIST 69

WHAT'S A PEDORTHIST? 69

Assessment 70

Formulation of a treatment 70

Implementation of the treatment plan.. 71

Follow-up treatment plan 71

ROCKER SHOES.. 73

STEEL SHANKS 75

CORTISONE INJECTIONS.. 76

NSAIDS 77

COUNTER-IRRITANTS 79

CAPSAICIN 79

SALICYLATES 80

LIDOCAINE PATCHES 80

"It is by faith that poetry, as well as devotion, soars above this dull earth; that imagination breaks through its clouds, breathes a purer air, and lives in a softer light." - Henry Giles

CHAPTER 1   LET ME START OUT BY SAYING

I wrote this book with one purpose in mind; To make sure no one (and I mean no one) need deal with sesamoiditis for months or years like I did. You and I are going to get through this problem. Had I known before what I know now, I would've saved myself a lot of aggravation, frustration, time and money!

This book will give you the information you need to understand sesamoiditis. I compiled the best and most current information into one book, in order to get you back into action as quickly as possible. I tried to be as comprehensive as possible so this book can serve as the one and only guide you'll ever need to deal with sesamoiditis.

What makes me an expert? I run. I run a lot. I also run far. I'm an engineer. Both of my parents are medical doctors (radiologists). I'm well versed in physiology, anatomy, kinesiology and I hate being injured. I also have flat arches in both my feet. I'm a prime candidate for sesamoiditis and I had to deal with it for over 2 years. I traveled around the country, specifically to see the top orthopedic surgeons, sports podiatrists, sports pedorthists, homeopaths and nutrionists. The information contained in this book is a compilation of everything I learned from doctors' visits and on my own. You may find pieces of this information on various websites in the same or different form, but you won't find all of the information contained in this book anywhere. It just isn't a high priority ailment and no one has written anything definitive on the subject.

Having an engineering-mind, I always want to break a system down and understand it from the inside-out. That's what this book's about. Your body is a system. Your foot is a feature of that system and if you have sesamoiditis, then there's a problem.

I've already done the leg-work. I've been the guinea pig. I've gone through trials and tribulations dealing with this. I've paid monies to see sports podiatrists, orthopedic surgeons, pedorthists, acupuncturists, acupressurists and physical therapists.

I did whatever it took to get back to being able to distance-run. I ran into quite a few road-blocks and problems. I made mistakes left and right, and had to deal with a lot of misinformation.

So, my hope is that this book will allow you to bypass all of that. I want you back in action just like I needed to be back in action. When you win, I win.

Let me first give you some background of what's physically going on and then I'll explain the solution.

As an aside, let me tell you how I got sesamoiditis. Like I said, I run a lot. I'm an endurance athlete. What does an endurance athlete do? I run hundred mile ultra-marathons. (Any running course over 26.2 miles is considered an ultra-marathon) The courses I run are some of the most grueling in the world. I trail run on mountains, at elevation, across many different kinds of landscapes. I'm always amazed at how hard some of the race courses actually are. Some are over 14,000 feet in elevation with jagged rock for miles.

That being said, in the last 4 years, even with all of the running I've done (over 200+ races), I've never had a foot problem whatsoever, not even a black toe or blister. I typically weigh around 225 pounds with a height of 6'4" and a 15 shoe size, so I'm clearly a likely candidate for problems as a runner. Nothing, nada, zilch in the way of foot problems.

There's a small mountain (a hill really) near where I live that I cross over multiple times in a workout session. Parts of the trail have sharp jagged rock and I'd try to run as much of it as possible. Some days I'd be out there for 5 hours non-stop, going up and down as fast as I could in 115-degree weather. It was this exercise, and mostly running the jagged rock, that eventually caused my sesamoiditis. Of all the courses I've run, this hill was one of the easiest ones, yet it was the one that took me out. How's that even possible? I don't know, but what I can tell you is, it happened. And the worst part was that I had no idea what sesamoiditis was. I'd never heard of it before. So what did I do? I ran through the pain and kept going. The worst thing you could possibly do.

This book should shed some light on why you can't out-smart a sesamoid injury and what you <u>can</u> do to get over this horrendous problem without making things worse.

It may seem a little odd that there's a section on your attitude. However, I believe that the reason people fail at anything, including curing themselves of ailments is because they lose hope <u>or</u> they don't follow through and do everything they need to do in order to fix the problem. If you're the alpha-type personality I am, maybe you don't need this attitude adjustment, and if not, feel free to skip that section. However, there is one undeniable fact to having the section and that is "It can't hurt".

Let's get this problem cured.

CHAPTER 2   AN ATTITUDE ADJUSTMENT

Before you start reading about sesamoiditis, the different modalities to combat it and my plan for curing it, let's talk about your attitude.

For some of you, you've had sesamoiditis for months or years at this point and you're tired of dealing with it. For others, you're athletes that can't stand to be sidelined with injury. For yet others, your job depends on you standing on your feet all day, as well as walking or having to carry heavy objects, all of which are terribly painful with sesamoiditis.

I receive emails all the time from people who are frantic because they're in so much pain. The problem just won't go away. And when I say frantic, some are actually suicidal. Everyone reacts differently, but if this issue is keeping you from something you need to do, I realize the enormity of the problem. If this is you, then I want you to use that emotion, use that energy, use your discontent to drive your staying on top of this problem. I promise, if you do that, you'll get to the other side of the problem sooner rather than later. It takes diligence, perseverance and dedication to overcome sesamoiditis.

Regardless of whether this is a new problem or one that's been around for a while, you must follow my instructions <u>exactly</u>. If you don't, your results may not be optimal.

Think of it like a combination lock. If you're off by just a little bit, or if you forget a number in the combination, or if you enter the numbers in the wrong order, the lock won't open. You'll only open this lock by using the exact combination I give you.

Maybe you don't like icing or don't think you have time for it. Maybe you believe acupuncture is hokey and won't bother trying it. Maybe you think you don't have the money for ultrasound. No matter what the excuse, that's all it is, an excuse. Excuses will get you nowhere. If you want results, you have to put in the time, effort and money. This book will help you minimize that burden.

So that being said, no excuses. Do exactly what I tell you in the order in which I prescribe. I don't care if you've already tried some of the things I write about. I'm sure you didn't do it in the exact manner and in the specific combination I prescribe, so give it another shot.

CHAPTER 3   WHAT ARE SESAMOIDS?

Generally speaking, a sesamoid is <u>any</u> bone embedded in a tendon. Sesamoids are found in several joints in the body.

In the normal foot, the sesamoids are two pea-shaped bones located in the ball of the foot beneath the big toe joint.

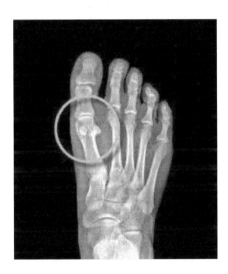

Acting as a pulley for tendons, the sesamoids help the big toe move normally and provide leverage when the big toe "pushes off" during walking and running. The sesamoids also serve as a weight-bearing surface for the first metatarsal bone (the long bone connected to the big toe), absorbing the weight placed on the ball of the foot when walking, running or jumping.

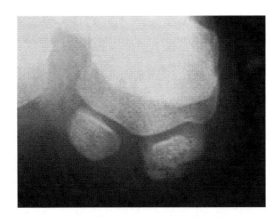

Sesamoid injuries can involve the bones, tendons, and/or surrounding tissue in the joint. They are often associated with activities requiring increased pressure on the ball of the foot, such as running, basketball, football, golf, tennis, and ballet. In addition, people with high arches are at risk for developing sesamoid problems. Frequent wearing of high-heeled shoes can also be a contributing factor.

CHAPTER 4   TYPES OF SESAMOID INJURIES IN THE FOOT

There are four diagnosis related to ball of foot pain revolving around sesamoiditis:

1. Turf toe: This is an injury of the soft tissue surrounding the big toe joint. It usually occurs when the big toe joint is extended beyond its normal range. Turf toe causes immediate, sharp pain and swelling. It usually affects the entire big toe joint and limits the motion of the toe. Turf toe may result in an injury to the soft tissue attached to the sesamoid or a fracture of the sesamoid. Sometimes a "pop" is felt at the moment of injury.

2. Fracture: A fracture (break) in a sesamoid bone can be either acute or chronic.

An acute fracture is caused by trauma – a direct blow or impact to the bone. An acute sesamoid fracture produces immediate pain and swelling at the site of the break, but usually does not affect the entire big toe joint.

A chronic fracture is a stress fracture (a hairline break usually caused by repetitive stress or overuse). A chronic sesamoid fracture produces longstanding pain in the ball of the foot beneath the big toe joint. The pain, which tends to come and go, generally is aggravated with activity and relieved with rest.

3. Sesamoiditis: This is an overuse injury involving chronic inflammation of the sesamoid bones and the tendons involved with those bones. Sesamoiditis is caused by increased pressure to the sesamoids. Often, sesamoiditis is associated with a dull, longstanding pain beneath the big toe joint. The pain comes and goes, usually occurring with certain shoes or certain activities.

CHAPTER 5   WHAT IS SESAMOIDITIS?

Simply put, sesamoiditis is inflammation of the sesamoid bones. In anatomy, a sesamoid bone is a bone embedded within a tendon.

Sesamoid bones can be found on joints throughout the body, including:

• In the knee — the patella (within the quadriceps tendon).

• In the hand — two sesamoid bones are commonly found in the distal portions of the first metacarpal bone (within the tendons of adductor pollicis and flexor pollicis brevis). There is also commonly a sesamoid bone in distal portions of the second metacarpal bone.

• In the wrist — The pisiform of the wrist is a sesamoid bone (within the tendon of flexor carpi ulnaris).

• In the foot — the first metatarsal bone usually has two sesamoid bones at its connection to the big toe (both within the tendon of flexor hallucis brevis). In some people, only a single sesamoid is found on the first MTP.

In humans (and animals like horses), it occurs on the bottom of the foot, just behind the large toe. There are normally two sesamoid bones on each foot. Sometimes sesamoids can be bipartite, which means they're comprised of two separate pieces. The sesamoids are roughly the size of small jelly beans.

The sesamoid bones act as a fulcrum for the flexor tendons, the tendons which bend the big toe downward.

Periostitis, also known as periostalgia, is a medical condition caused by inflammation of the periosteum, a layer of connective tissue that surrounds bone. The condition is generally chronic, and is marked by tenderness and swelling of the bone and an aching pain.

Usually periostitis occurs along with sesamoiditis, and the suspensory ligament may also be affected. This periostitis can actually be the cause of inflammation in the area once it occurs.

Osteophytes or new bone with jagged edges can form that push on the tendon in such a way as to cause inflammation as well. Once this occurs, the problem may be chronic. This is very important for you to understand as you'll later read in this book.

Inflammation, in most cases, is not your friend and must be treated vehemently.

In summary, sesamoiditis results in inflammation, pain, and eventually bone growth directly in the area of the sesamoids.

In addition to experiencing inflammation and pain, the sesamoid bone may fracture and can be difficult to pick up on x-ray. A bone scan is a better alternative.

Make sure you understand the distinction between x-ray and a bone scan because you'll want to be well versed in these technologies if you see a doctor.

Most podiatrists will just take an x-ray, which in most cases is relatively inaccurate. Why do they take an x-ray? Maybe for insurance reasons, costs or because they don't have a bone scan machine. Either way, choose a provider whose able to do a bone scan if necessary.

What is a bone scan?

A bone scan is a test to help find the cause of your foot pain. It is done to find damage to the bones, find cancer that has spread to the bones or to follow problems such as infection and trauma to the bones. A bone scan can often find a problem - days to months earlier than a regular x-ray test.

For a bone scan, a radioactive substance is injected into a vein in your arm. This substance, called a tracer, travels through your bloodstream and into your bones. This could take several hours.

A special camera takes pictures of the tracer in your bones. Areas that absorb little or no amount of tracer appear as dark or "cold" spots. This could show a lack of blood supply to the bone or certain types of cancer.

Areas of fast bone growth or repair absorb more tracer and show up as bright or "hot" spot in the pictures. Hot spots may point to problems such as arthritis, a tumor, a fracture, or an infection.

CHAPTER 6   CAUSES OF SESAMOIDITIS

Sesamoiditis is usually caused by repetitive, excessive pressure on the forefoot. It typically develops when the structures of the first metatarsophalangeal joint are subjected to chronic pressure and tension. The surrounding tissues respond by becoming irritated and inflamed. This is a common problem among ballet dancers, people who work on their feet all day and athletes who play any kind of sport that puts excessive pressure on the forefoot area. Any activity that places constant force on the ball of the foot—even walking—can cause sesamoiditis.

Trauma to the sesamoid bone may result in sesamoiditis. Stress fractures (microscopic tears in the bone structure due to repetitive abuse) can produce this condition.

Sesamoiditis can also be an overuse injury that involves chronic, or long-term, inflammation of your sesamoid bones and the tendons that act on these bones. In most cases, a sudden and excessive upward bending force on your big toe causes sesamoiditis, although wearing high heels and experiencing certain types of foot trauma may also contribute to your sesamoiditis.

Conventional footwear plays an important role in aggravating your sesamoids and surrounding structures. Shoes with tapered toe boxes and toe-spring can cause sesamoids to become dislocated, causing dysfunction.

When your hallux, or big toe, is properly aligned with your first metatarsal bone, your sesamoids are also properly aligned and function as intended.

Sesamoiditis commonly involve a dull pain under your big toe joint that fails to resolve over time. Some sesamoiditis-related pain is usually intermittent, or comes and goes, and may be worse when wearing certain shoes or participating in certain activities.

CHAPTER 7   SYMPTOMS OF SESAMOIDITIS

Sesamoiditis typically can be distinguished from other conditions that cause pain in the forefoot by its gradual onset. The foot pain usually begins as a mild ache and increases gradually, if you continue the aggravating activity. It may build to an intense throbbing.

In most cases, sesamoiditis causes little to no bruising or redness. Pain and swelling can limit the ability of the first metatarsophalangeal joint to flex upward (dorsiflexion) or downward (plantarflexion), causing loss of range of motion in the big toe and difficulty walking.

Some of the most common signs and symptoms associated with sesamoiditis include:

• Pain focused under the big toe on the ball of the foot.

• Pain in the affected area that develops gradually.

• Swelling and bruising.

• Impaired ability to bend or straighten the big toe.

CHAPTER 8   THE DIAGNOSIS OF SESAMOIDITIS

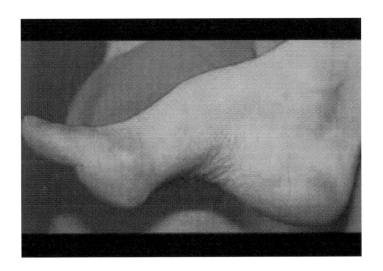

During the examination, the physician will look for tenderness at the sesamoid bones. Your doctor may manipulate the bone slightly or ask you to bend and straighten the toe. He or she may also bend the great toe up toward the top of the foot to see if pain intensifies.

Your physician will request x-rays (even though a bone scan is more appropriate) of the forefoot to ensure a proper diagnosis. In many people, the sesamoid bone nearer the center of the foot (the medial sesamoid) has two parts (bipartite). Because the edges of a bipartite medial sesamoid are generally smooth, and the edges of a fractured sesamoid are generally jagged, an x-ray can be useful in making an appropriate diagnosis.

Again a bone scan is a more accurate test. Your physician may also request x-rays of the other foot to compare the bone structure. This is the best way for the physician to determine if what he's seeing in one foot is normal, by comparing the look of the sesamoid to the other foot. If the x-rays appear normal and pain continues, the physician may request a bone scan.

CHAPTER 9   THE "USUAL" TREATMENT OF SESAMOIDITIS

This section details the current method for treatment of sesamoiditis. I'll assume you haven't talked to a doctor or done your own research yet. This section will discuss what to expect from a doctor's visit.

Sesamoiditis treatment is generally non-operative. However, if conservative measures fail, your physician may recommend surgery to remove the sesamoid bone. Surgery should be a last resort if you're an athlete. Surgery can sometimes cause different issues that are just as bad as having sesamoiditis.

Treatment protocol for sesamoiditis

1. Stop the activity causing the pain.
2. Take aspirin or NSAID's (ibuprofen for example) to relieve the pain. A weekly regimen of 800mg of ibuprofen 4 times a day for 7 days to begin with or 1 325 mg aspirin every 12 hours is optimal. (Make sure your provider is aware of your medication use before starting any regimen.)

3. Rest and ice the sole of your foot. Do not apply ice directly to the skin, but use an ice pack or wrap the ice in a towel.

4. Wear soft-soled, low-heeled shoes. Stiff-soled shoes like clogs may also be comfortable.

5. Use a felt cushioning pad to relieve stress.

6. Return to activity gradually and continue to wear a cushioning pad of dense foam rubber under the sesamoids to support them. Avoid activities that put weight on the balls of the feet.

7. Tape the great toe so that it remains bent slightly downward (plantar flexion).

8. Your doctor may recommend an injection of a steroid medication to reduce swelling.

9. If symptoms persist, you may need to wear a removable short leg fracture brace for 4 to 6 weeks. Injured or inflamed sesamoid bones can be difficult to heal, because you almost continuously put pressure on these structures every time you stand or walk. Conservative care methods may be helpful in resolving your sesamoiditis.

Conservative treatment techniques include:

Shoe therapy: Footwear that allows proper toe splay can help. Toe splay can be enabled with a toe spacing device.

Immobilization: Your affected foot may be placed in a cast or removable walking cast to help rest the injured or irritated tissues. Crutches can help reduce the amount of force on the sesamoids.

Taping or strapping: Your involved toe may be taped or strapped to help reduce tension on the sesamoid bones.

Padding: A special pad may be placed inside your shoe to help cushion the sesamoid bones. A metatarsal pad helps return the fat pad in the ball of your foot to a place where it will protect your sesamoids.

Physical therapy (PT): PT is an important treatment measure, especially following immobilization. Range-of-motion exercises and ultrasound therapy are among the most commonly used PT modalities for sesamoiditis.

Anti-inflammatory medication, cortisone injections, and certain types of surgery are more aggressive treatment measures for treating sesamoiditis and may be necessary in some individuals.

Again, a doctor may recommend surgery, including sesamoid bone removal, if conservative care measures fail to resolve the problem.

CHAPTER 10 SESAMOID FRACTURE, A SLIGHTLY DIFFERENT BEAST

A sesamoid fracture of one or both sesamoid bones produces many of the same symptoms as sesamoiditis: pain in the ball of the foot and first metatarsophalangeal joint, swelling, and limited plantarflexion/dorsiflexion.

In sesamoiditis, chronic abuse causes a gradual onset of pain. The onset of pain with a sesamoid fracture is from traumatic injury to the ball of the foot. This commonly involves a fall from height, in which the patient lands heavily on the foot, fracturing one or both sesamoid bones.

A fractured sesamoid produces substantial swelling throughout the forefoot and a deep, tender bruise in the area of the big toe's metatarsophalangeal joint. X-rays or bone scans are often necessary to confirm a sesamoid fracture. Occasionally, x-rays are inconclusive because a small percentage of people have bipartite sesamoid bones. Instead of one medial and one lateral sesamoid bone under each first metatarsal head, some people have sesamoid bones that are divided into two pieces (You're born this way). Because these bones are so small, radiologists may be unable to distinguish a fractured sesamoid from a bipartite sesamoid, or a fractured bipartite sesamoid from a whole one. In rare cases, a bone scan may be necessary to confirm a fracture.

Treatment for a sesamoid fracture involves keeping the injured foot completely immobilized without <u>any</u> weight bearing for 6 to 8 weeks. The first metatarsophalangeal joint must be fully immobilized. If pain persists in the forefoot after 8 weeks of treatment or if joint function is not restored in the first metatarsophalangeal joint, removal of the sesamoid bone(s) (a sesamoidectomy) may be necessary. This procedure is a last resort, because removal of one or both sesamoid bones, or damage to the surrounding soft tissue structures can severely compromise normal foot function.

For example, surgically removing the medial sesamoid requires an incision along the inner side of the big toe's metatarsophalangeal joint. Cutting these tissues may damage the joint capsule, resulting in weakness and misalignment of the metatarsal-phalangeal joint and lead to the development of a bunion.

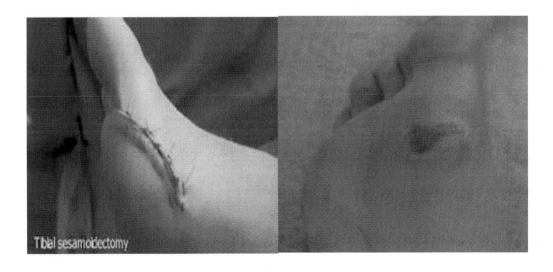

Tibial sesamoidectomy

A bunion is a bulge or bump that develops on the side of the foot, near the base of the big toe. Physicians call this deformity hallux abducto valgus or HAV, meaning the hallux turns away (abducts) from the midline of the foot and twists so the inside edge touches the ground and the outside edge turns upward. Essentially, it's the big toe's tendency to point to the outside of the foot. The condition worsens over time, causing discomfort, pain, skin problems (e.g., corns and lesions), and difficulty walking.

Treatment for a Sesamoid Fracture

• You will need to wear a stiff-soled shoe or a short leg-fracture brace.

• Your physician may tape the joint to limit movement of the great toe.

• You may have to wear a J-shaped pad around the area of the sesamoid to relieve pressure as the fracture heals.

• Pain relievers such as aspirin or NSAID's may be recommended.

• Generally, it may take several months for the discomfort to subside.

• Cushioning pads or other orthotic devices are often helpful as the fracture heals.

If you have a fracture, it must heal before you can begin any kind of therapy whatsoever. I can't stress this enough. As long as the fracture is present, you must stay off of the foot.

CHAPTER 11 THE FIRST THING YOU NEED TO DO

You may need to read this section several times. The information contained here is extremely important.

Stop causing <u>any</u> inflammation whatsoever to the sesamoid area, as well as the big toe joint. This is everything. Let me repeat, this is everything.

The reason why sesamoiditis is such a pain in the ass is because once the area is inflamed, it's very difficult for blood to get into the tiny sesamoid fissures that allow the sesamoids to heal. Each pea-sized sesamoid has a very tiny canal that carries blood into the bone. By design, It's already very difficult for blood to travel into these canals as it is. The design was poor but who are we going to complain to? Just know that this problem is compounded when <u>any</u> inflammation occurs in the area.

It's crucial you get rid of the existing inflammation as well as stop any additional inflammation caused by pressure to the area. Walking or standing in place is the worst thing one can do. A walking motion actually uses the big toe <u>more</u> than jogging. If you jog with a mid-foot or heel-strike, you're doing just that, you're taking all the pressure off of the forefoot. Unfortunately, when we walk or stand for long periods of time we actually put more pressure on the forefoot and hence more pressure on the sesamoid area. This is a huge problem. Alright so what do I do? Read on.

CHAPTER 12 A SUMMARY OF WHAT WE'RE DEALING WITH

The following is a brief summary of all the components that come into play when dealing with most forms of sesamoiditis.

• The sesamoid bones themselves have been damaged and are causing pain.

• The periosteum between the tendon and sesamoid bones are chronically inflamed and causing pain.

• Osteophytes have developed and are causing inflammation and pain in the area.

• Bending of the big toe joint is causing stress, pain and swelling in the area.

• Inflammation in the general forefoot area is causing additional pain, swelling and making it harder for the sesamoiditis to heal.

• Arthritis in the big toe joint is very common and can be the cause of pain, swelling and discomfort. An x-ray or bone scan should determine if arthritic changes have occurred.

It's important to address each and every issue, because problems will continue if you fail to address any one issue.

CHAPTER 13 STEP BY STEP GUIDE TO BEATING SESAMOIDITIS

Here's my step-by-step procedure to guide you through exactly what you need to do at the onset of sesamoiditis. This guide is the same for any gradation of sesamoiditis, with the exception of fracture. (Fractures must heal before beginning treatments!)

For non-fracture sesamoiditis

Step 1 - Stop causing pain and inflammation to your forefoot.

• Initially, keep walking or standing to a minimum.

• Take a picture from a side angle of your foot, being sure to capture the ball of the foot so as to have a basis for future comparison. We manage what we measure.

• Make sure you're wearing shoes loosely.

• Wear tennis or walking shoes at all times. The more rigid the sole of the shoe the better.

• Keep bending of the big toe to a minimum.

• Do not wear high heel shoes or dress shoes with zero padding.

• When you sit in a chair, don't put pressure on your forefoot. Pressure will cause swelling and inflammation.

Step 2 – Know what you are dealing with.

If the ball of your foot looks enlarged, it's inflamed and is a possible indication of sesamoid fracture.

As a side note; a lot of people are actually born with abnormally shaped sesamoids in their feet, so without a baseline for comparison, a doctor may not know if what he/she is seeing on an x-ray or bone scan is normal for you. The best indicator of whether the sesamoid bones are normal in one foot is to x-ray or bone scan the other foot for comparison. This is still not a great indicator.

That being said, there are obvious signs of trauma and fracture that doctors should be able to see if the problem's bad enough.

If you have inflammation, you need to determine whether or not you're dealing with a fracture right away.

What type of doctor should you see for sesamoiditis?

Find a "sports" podiatrist. A regular podiatrist might work but a "sports" podiatrist typically has more exposure to problems like sesamoiditis. This will save you time and money.

What about an orthopedic surgeon - foot specialist?

Yes, you can see this type of doctor, but I generally find the sports podiatrist to be a better fit and more cost effective. Most surgeons are naturally inclined to recommend a more aggressive treatment that you may not need. If you do opt to see an orthopaedic surgeon, be sure to see a foot specialist. They'll have more experience with this type of condition.

This is probably a good time to bring up the fact that under no circumstances do you want to get a "sesamoidectomy" unless everything else fails. I can't stress enough how bad your condition has to be to have a sesamoidectomy. After living with sesamoiditis for over 8 months, I almost gave up and just said "The hell with it, I'm getting a double sesamoidectomy" which would have been a huge mistake based on all the research and feedback I've gotten.

Why shouldn't I have a sesamoidectomy?

The sesamoidectomy, once done, ruins the integrity of how you walk, run and even balance on your foot. There are no guarantees the sesamoidectomy will not make things worse. This is especially true if you're an athlete and depend on your forefoot for more than just leisurely walking.

It's true that some people have reported their pain subsided after about a year of recovery, but the positive reports are few and far between. Depending on your age, recovery from a sesamoidectomy conservatively will take at least a year, if it's going to happen at all.

Step 3 - Stop additional damage

You must take all pressure off the sesamoid area as well as stop any upward bending of the big toe. This is where big toe taping comes in. This is where having the correct orthotic in your shoe comes in. The correct orthotic will change the arch of your foot in such a way as to take pressure off the ball of the foot. A proper orthotic usually has a trough area or gouge where the ball of the foot lays, in order to keep it from a normal impact during a foot strike. This is very important and will make an immediate and substantial impact on the amount of inflammation present.

Step 4 - Get rid of inflammation

You must rid the ball of foot of any existing inflammation as well as pain. Massage after a treatment of acupuncture and ultrasound is a great way to break up any new bone (bone spurs) that may have accumulated in the area.

Step 5 – Make sure the problem is gone before you do things normally

Make sure <u>all</u> of the inflammation and pain has completely subsided. Do little tests with your foot, testing for pain, before going back to normal activity.

Why is this important? Because once you've had sesamoiditis the forefoot area is forever weakened and prone to re-injury.

The last thing you want to do is start any type of activity without the correct shoes and orthotics. You'll just have to start over again.

You can test whether or not a problem still exists in a few ways:

• Walk barefoot on hard concrete in a normal fashion and see if there's any pain at all.

• Do some forefoot pushups. In other words, lean up against a wall and lift yourself with your forefoot onto your tippy toes and see whether or not this produces any kind of pain. (Be careful)

• With a bare foot, use your hands to put pressure on the sesamoid area rather firmly to determine if any pain still exists.

If you have any pain at all, in the ball of your foot, don't resume normal activity. If you do resume normal activity, you'll lose the benefit of any treatment you've done up until this point.

The following treatment plan should be followed immediately.

Preparation

Your bed: Elevate your foot or feet while you sleep at night. Inflammation in the legs and feet happens rather dramatically when sleeping on a flat bed. Take a thick pillow or pillows and put them between the box-spring and the mattress of the bed to elevate the end of your mattress. The goal is to have your feet elevated above your heart all night long.

Next to your bed: Keep a pair of flat rigid sandals or tennis shoes, with orthotics in them, so you don't step on hard floor upon getting out of bed. Any walking at all will cause damage and inflammation. Immediately put your feet into a shoe when getting out of bed.

In your freezer: Always have ice packs or freeze water in small paper cups as you'll be icing your forefoot area often.

The Plan

Start supplementing with calcium citrate. Calcium is very important for bones to heal properly and to avoid the formation of osteophytes (bone spurs).

As soon as you wake up, ice the ball of your foot. You'd be amazed at how much inflammation happens when you sleep at night when lying flat. Ice the area for exactly 20 minutes, no more, no less.

Massage the forefoot immediately after icing. You'll want to do this for about 5 minutes and do it rather firmly. It may be painful but the point is to break up or disallow any newly formed bone in the area. Massage also helps promote blood into the area. (Do not press too hard.)

Ice the foot again, in four hours, for another twenty minutes. If you have foot pain in other parts of your foot, due to avoiding pressure on the ball of your foot, (walking on the outer edge of your foot) I recommend getting a plastic bucket that's big enough for your foot (or feet), fill it with ice and water and submerse your entire foot in it. Soaking your foot in ice water works wonders for reducing inflammation.

Ice about an hour before you go to bed. The reason for this is because you've most likely caused inflammation in the foot due to walking. Gravity from standing will cause inflammation in the feet as well. You don't want to go to bed with inflammation.

For most, NSAIDS (nonsteroidals) are your friend. Begin taking a regimen of whatever NSAID works best for you. I personally take ibuprofen and follow a two-week regimen of diminishing dosages. i.e. Take 800mg per day, 4 times a day (every 6 hours) for 1 week. Then lower the dosage to 600mg per day, 4 times a day for the next week. Please consult your doctor if you are unsure about taking NSAID's.

For those of you who can't take an NSAID and would prefer natural alternatives, try Tumeric. Tumeric actually works fairly well at high dosages to hedge against inflammation. You can buy Tumeric on amazon.com or at your local health food store.

For the first two weeks (6 treatments, 3 per week), you'll do the following every other day:

• Acupuncture for up to 40 minutes in and around the forefoot area.

• Ultrasound for up to 15 minutes immediately following the acupuncture.

• Massage the ball of your foot and big toe joint for about 5 minutes, immediately after the ultrasound. Be somewhat aggressive here but again not too hard to cause trauma to the area. You want to break up any scar tissue or additional bone growth that has occurred.

• As soon as possible, get in to see a pedorthist. Explain to the pedorthist exactly what the problem is and that you need an orthotic specifically made for sesamoiditis. Have him/her recommend what shoe to wear given your type of feet. (High arch, low arch, etc.)

Repeat this regimen after two weeks if your pain isn't substantially better. Allow at least two weeks before starting acupuncture and ultrasound again. Overdoing these modalities could make the area worse.

CHAPTER 14 THE ROLE OF NUTRITION AND CALCIUM

Nutrition plays a large role in the healing process. It may also have played a role in how you got injured in the first place. Either way, some adjustments to your diet may help expedite the healing process.

Nutrition is so important that I've dedicated an entire chapter to it. Implement everything you read in this chapter to help speed up the healing process. You may need to read this chapter a few times.

Normally, specialized cells called "osteoblasts" add fresh minerals (primarily calcium, but others, too) to bone and "osteoclasts" remove older bone tissue by properly breaking down the minerals and reabsorbing them into the bloodstream. Both processes are intricately interlinked and crucial for health. But they must be supported with the right nutrients, and this is where we usually fall short.

In cases where bone spurs form as a correction to weakened bone structure, you'll want to rid yourself of the bone spurs while still building healthy bones with the right diet and supplementation.

That's one of the odd things about calcium in the body. It doesn't always build up where we'd like it to. So, while weak bones can lead to the development of bone spurs, you'll still need ingredients to dissolve this unwanted bone.

At other times, lifestyle, genetics, or a combination of both, conspire to create bone spurs. In this case, your individual pH may tend toward a more alkaline nature, setting the pieces in place for calcium to build up where you don't want it.

The strange thing about developing bone spurs, and the connection to pH, is that most people's diets are so acidic that the body has a tough time keeping things equal and close to a "7" on the pH scale. But it can – and clearly does – happen nonetheless.

That's one of the reasons why pH can be such a deciding factor.

To function at its best, the body must maintain a proper and delicate acid/alkaline (pH) balance. An over-alkaline system makes calcium harder to absorb, and calcium is essential for strengthening bones. So, once load-bearing bones are under a lot of stress, they try out some "quick fixes" to shore up against the added pressure. One of fixes happens to be growth of bone spurs.

To begin with, the standard American diet is very much to blame for the development of weak bones, bone spurs, and kidney stones. Contributing foods and ingredients include high-fructose corn syrup, soda, apple juice, fluoridated water, and other refined sugars. Combine that with the fact that most people don't hydrate enough during the day, and you have a "perfect storm" of conditions.

Of course, people who are very active can get bone spurs as a result of repetitive activity (like running, pitching or carpentry), and the irritation, pain, and stiffness they feel might not just be muscle aches but actual change in the structure of their joints. In these cases, bone spurs can appear in the shoulders where bones, muscles, and ligaments wear against each other, and in the heels, which take a lot of punishment from exercise, work and everyday life.

Even fashion can play a role. Shoes that are too tight and restrict the movement of the tendons can damage the bones of the feet. The bones of the bottom of the feet, called the "plantar surface" are covered with a tough fibrous tissue called the "fascia". This tissue stretches under the feet, and as you would guess (or have even experienced), can become damaged and inflamed, a condition called "plantar fasciitis." This essentially muscle-based damage can be the first step in developing heel spurs, because in the course of trying to repair damage to the feet, extra "emergency" bone can develop, becoming a spur of unwanted – and potentially debilitating – calcium.

You may not realize you have a bone spur until it begins to restrict movement and becomes painful. After all, 1 in 10 people have heel spurs, yet it can take years to notice. But when they do become painful, you'll want them gone, fast.

While some bone spurs can be identified by palpation, you may not determine the truth until you get your foot x-rayed. At that point, your conventional options are limited to non-steroidal anti-inflammatory drugs (NSAIDs) like ibuprofen or prescriptions, or possibly invasive and potentially complicated surgery.

Aside from being uncomfortable and restricting mobility, bone spurs can also break off and "float" in the joint, or become stuck in cushioning synovial fluid between the joints, which can be both debilitating and painful.

Bone spurs can happen to anyone, and whatever your situation, the ingredients I recommend will help. These ingredients don't affect healthy bones. Bone spurs develop where there's injury, poor blood supply, scar tissue or some other damage. In a sense, it's truly "dead bone." The formula I recommend only breaks down this dead bone. It will not dissolve or harm healthy bone.

The Ingredients that can help

Ammonium chloride sounds like a potentially scary thing, but it's not. It's absolutely essential in helping support the normal growth cycle of bones. It's mildly acidic and can help the body return to a healthy acid/alkaline balance. It's actually a component of our digestive juices and stomach acid, and is crucial for mineral absorption.

Calcium chloride: There are many forms of calcium around. As you might have guessed, the calcium I recommend in this case isn't for building up bone as much as it is for helping keep the overall bone resorption process running smoothly. Calcium phosphate – another form of calcium, and the same kind found in our bones and teeth – is an additional ingredient I recommend for this formula. Remember, almost all of the calcium in our bodies is used to create healthy bones. So you don't want to cut calcium from your diet and supplement regimen in order to fight bone spurs. In fact, you're much more likely to develop bone spurs without appropriate calcium intake.

Betaine Hydrochloric acid is another acidifying ingredient that mimics the stomach acid we create naturally to help break down minerals properly. In an over-alkaline environment where calcium and other minerals aren't prepared for the body to absorb well, you'll see the formation of bone spurs, calcium deposits, and kidney stones. As calcium crystals collect at the site of an injury or weak bone, a bone spur is certain to follow.

Vitamin C is generally considered an immune booster, but vitamin C is crucial for collagen formation during the tissue rebuilding phase after injury or other heavy activity. Any deficiency of vitamin C doesn't just slow down this process, but actually weakens ligaments and tendons. So it's essential to keep the cushioning and connective tissue of our joints healthy so the body doesn't overcompensate by creating bone spurs. Plus, vitamin C fights the oxidative stress that can hinder joint repair—another reason to include it in your regimen.

Vitamin B6 as P-5-P: The P-5-P (pyridoxal-5-phosphate) form of vitamin B6 is readily absorbed by the body and doesn't need to be converted by the liver. It's a perfect nutrient to combine with magnesium (in this case, magnesium glycerophosphate, an acidic form) to help ensure proper calcium absorption and use by the body. After all, you're still getting calcium from your diet and supplement regimen while you're getting rid of bone spurs (and that's a good thing.) You just want to make sure that the calcium you get stays fluid and doesn't form into the clumps that can cause kidney stones or improper build up at the joints. Since P-5-P works so well with magnesium, a key ingredient for proper bone building, it's definitely one you want to have on board.

Magnesium glycerophosphate: Magnesium is one of the most important minerals in our lives, and one that is often missing from our diets. That's because many of our soils are so mineral depleted that any magnesium that should be present in foods usually isn't.

Magnesium helps our cells build energy, assists calcium in bone-building, and helps relieve pain by blocking a pain receptor called the NMDA receptor. The glycerophosphate form is the type I recommend for this use because it is the acidic form of the mineral, so it will not alkalinize body tissues, and potentially add to the problem of bone spurs.

Source: http://www.terrytalksnutrition.com

CHAPTER 15 A COMPREHENSIVE LIST OF MODALITIES

The following is a comprehensive list of everything that will help treat sesamoiditis. I've personally used every single one of these. While some worked better than others, remember, you're not me and your problem and foot issues are unique to you. That means that some of these may work better or worse for you than they did for me. It's important to understand that you may not just have sesamoiditis. You may have a combination of issues with your foot, so it's important to address all of the issues and not just the sesamoiditis.

Regardless of your foot issues, this list will cover a lot of the same treatment modalities for a plethora of foot problems. The key is to be consistent and persistent.

Please note that it's outside the scope of this book to determine duration, frequency or even whether using a particular modality is right for you and your condition. You may want to consult a doctor.

Calcium

Calcium is the most abundant mineral in the body but may also be the most deficient. The amount of calcium that we absorb from our food varies widely. Our age is one factor. An adolescent may absorb up to 75% of the calcium obtained from foods, while in adults the maximum absorption rate ranges from 20% to 30%.

Even though our bones feel solid and seem permanent they're just like any other body tissue - they're constantly being broken down and formed again. In an adult, 20 percent of bone calcium is withdrawn from bones and replaced each year. Thus, every five years the bones are renewed.

Calcium is found in the extra cellular fluids and soft tissues of the body where it is vital to normal cell functioning. Much of the calcium in soft tissues is concentrated in muscle, although it is contained in the membrane and cytoplasm of every cell.

When the body is deficient of calcium it begins to leach calcium from the bones. In many people this happens to be in the heel of the foot or some other weak area of the body. As the calcium is being leached, it forms an eruption (similar to a volcano). This eruption is the bone spur.

Many people that have suffered from bone spurs found relief when they properly supplemented their diet daily with "good" calcium. They found that providing their body with "good" calcium along with other vital minerals stopped the "leaching process" (calcium deficiency) thus allowing the bone spur to shrink down and eventually disappear. With the bone spur gone, the surrounding damage from the spur is able to heal also.

Source: http://www.bonespur.com

Acupuncture

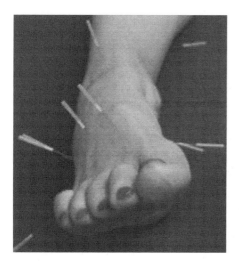

Acupuncture can be a touchy subject for some people. Most have probably never tried acupuncture for any reason. For some, it conjures thoughts of hippies or weirdo's or god knows what when you think of acupuncture and it would never cross your mind to try it. I'm here to tell you acupuncture does wonders for <u>some</u> medical issues. I'm not going to debate whether or not acupuncture works for anything more than muscle and tendon inflammation, because that's all we really care about here. You'll see noticeable differences literally overnight when following an acupuncture regimen.

Acupuncture is key to reducing the original inflammation, as well as hedging against future inflammation.

Acupuncture usually costs anywhere from $0 to $100 per session, with the average being around $45 per session. You can get acupuncture for next to nothing if you search for deals on sites like www.groupon.com.

Acupuncture with E-STIM

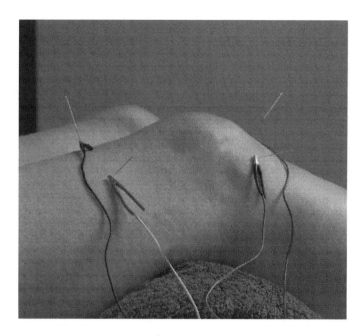

Acupuncture with electrical stimulation (E-STIM) works extremely well for muscle and tendon inflammation, sometimes better than dry needling does.

Electroacupuncture is a form of acupuncture where a small electric current is passed between pairs of acupuncture needles. According to some acupuncturists, this practice augments the use of regular acupuncture and is particularly good for treating pain and inflammation.

There are plenty of articles and research that conclude this form of acupuncture to have no merit, but I assure you there is a noticeable effect on the area. You'll see the difference within 24 hours.

Icing, bag of ice, straps, Dixie cup

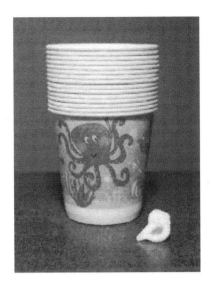

There are many different ways to deliver cold to an area. When we talk about icing, that ice can be delivered by using ice in a Ziploc bag, ice in a grocery bag or ice packs you can strap onto your body with Velcro. As far as sesamoiditis is concerned, if you don't have access to an ice foot bath (bucket with ice and water) then the best method of cold delivery will be to buy small paper cups, fill them with water and freeze them. What does this do? This allows you to rub the sesamoid and big toe joint area in concentric circles directly. When the ice melts, peel some of the paper off to expose more ice to continue icing the area. This works much better than a bag of ice.

Foot ice baths using a storage container

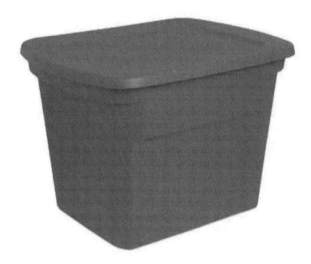

Most people hate taking ice baths. All we need to do is get your feet ankle high submersed in ice water. This is one of the most effective ways to treat sesamoiditis for a number of reasons. The main reason is that foot ice bath works wonders on reducing inflammation, not only in the sesamoid area, but all over your foot.

Why are full foot ice-baths so important? Because sesamoid pain will change your gait as well as your actual natural foot strike. You'll begin to put pressure on areas of your foot you don't normally put pressure on, and that will cause pain and inflammation in other areas of your foot. This method of cold delivery will not only help the sesamoid area, but will also help inflammation across the entire foot.

The best way to deal with entire foot inflammation is to buy a storage container from a store like Walmart or amazon.com big enough to fit your feet and deep enough to fill the container at least ankle high with ice and water. This is the runner's best friend. I use this all the time regardless of whether or not I'm injured.

Instead of using ice cubes, go to a convenience store and get a big plastic cup, preferably 64 ounces, fill it with water and freeze it. You can dump one big ice block into the container.

Taping the big toe down

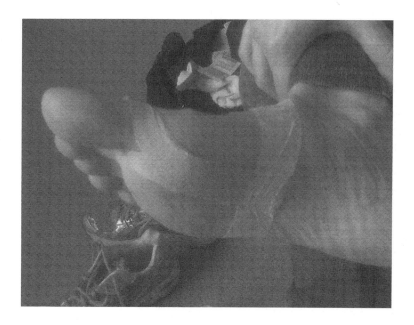

Taping the big toe down is extremely important because part of sesamoiditis has to do with putting pressure directly on the sesamoid bone, but another part of sesamoiditis is allowing the big toe to bend upwards, which causes stress on the joint and hence inflammation and pain. If you do anything that allows the big toe to flex up, it'll be very difficult to get rid of sesamoiditis. See the picture above which details exactly how you should tape your foot. Taping the foot may not feel like it's doing much, but it does make a world of difference. I highly recommend this.

Shoelaces

There are shoelaces and then there are shoelaces. It's important to wear shoes very loosely by tying your laces very loosely. When shoes are on tight, they're going to put too much pressure on the foot, including the forefoot area. This will cause swelling and inflammation. I recommend you get no lace shoelaces which are flexible and look like small bungee cords. They give your foot plenty of flex inside the shoe and allow for the shoe to "give" if your feet have swelled from running or standing. An example of tie-less shoe laces are "Nathan Shoe Lock Laces" which can be found in most shoe stores or on the web.

Das Boot! (The Boot!)

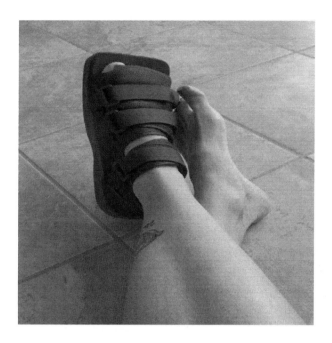

Some doctors will suggest wearing a boot to immobilize your foot when there is fracture or sesamoiditis is chronic. The boot does two primary things that help reduce inflammation: It keeps the pressure off the sesamoid area and it keeps the big toe from flexing.

Are you starting to see a recurring theme here? Do not put pressure on the sesamoid area and do not flex the big toe at all when walking. There are other ways to accomplish this, but if you don't mind wearing the boot, it will definitely work well. You may have to wear the boot for weeks depending on what other modalities you choose to use in order to treat the sesamoiditis.

Dancer Pads

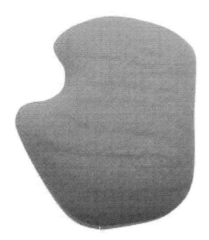

Dancer pads are so named because sesamoiditis was very common in ballet dancers who put a lot of pressure on their forefoot while dancing. This type of pad either fits inside the shoe loosely or adheres to the bottom of the shoe. The dancer pad works well for some and not so well for others, depending on how much inflammation you have in the area. If you have a lot of inflammation, the dancer pad won't be thick enough to relieve the pressure on the sesamoid area. Dancer pads work best when you've already reduced most of the inflammation to the area.

Sesamoid Wrap

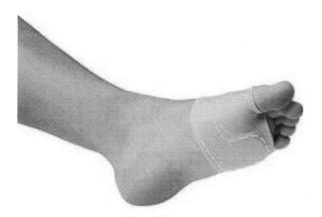

The sesamoid wrap works just like the dancer pad, only you wear it like a sock on the foot. This wrap works just as well, if not better than the dancer pad and stays in place. It is also typically washable. Again, this will not be very effective if the size of the ball of your foot is larger than the thickness of the pad inside the wrap. If the ball of your foot is still hitting the ground when you walk, and pressure is being exerted on the sesamoid area, this will not work well.

Metatarsal Pads

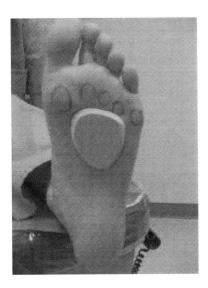

Metatarsal pads work a little different than sesamoid pads and are not necessarily used for sesamoiditis but can work wonders regardless. The metatarsal pad moves the foot strike lower on the foot so little to no pressure is put on the entire forefoot, not just the sesamoid area. These pads are usually thicker then dancer pads, so if the ball of your foot is inflamed, this may initially work better for you then the dancer pad. I used a combination of the metatarsal pad as well as a dancer pad which seemed to work well for me. You can also double up on these pads as long as it doesn't create discomfort when you walk.

Felt padding

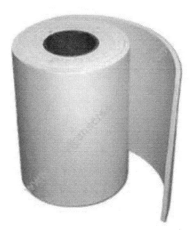

You can buy felt padding in rolls on amazon.com or at any number of websites on the internet. Felt padding is great for creating your own custom metatarsal pads or dancer pads. It will allow you to custom fit your foot exactly. You can also double up on the felt to raise your forefoot to disallow pressure on the ball of your foot when walking.

TENS device

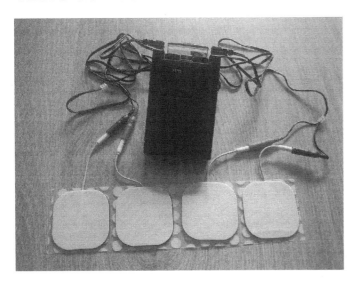

Transcutaneous electrical nerve stimulation (TENS) is the use of electric current produced by a device to stimulate the muscles, tendons and nerves for therapeutic purposes. TENS by definition covers the complete range of transcutaneously applied currents used for nerve excitation although the term is often used with a more restrictive intent, namely to describe the kind of pulses produced by portable stimulators used to treat pain. The unit is usually connected to the skin using two or more electrodes. A typical battery-operated TENS unit is able to modulate pulse width, frequency and intensity. Generally, TENS is applied at high frequency (>50 Hz) with an intensity below motor contraction (sensory intensity) or low frequency (<10 Hz) with an intensity that produces motor contraction.

Using a TENS device directly on the ball of the foot will help stimulate blood flow into the area. Some people will tell you that this is meant for muscle and not useful in situations like sesamoiditis but I disagree. It does work and you'll see the effects of within 24 hours. Be sure to ice right after you're done using this device. Use the TENS device for <u>no</u> longer than 10 minutes in a session and make sure you just barely feel the current in the ball of your foot. You can do damage if you turn the electrical current up too high.

You can buy a TENS device on amazon.com or other websites on the internet.

Ultrasound

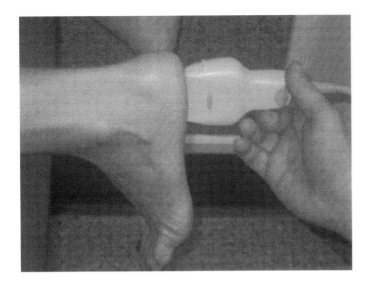

Using ultrasound in conjunction with acupuncture is one of the very best defenses against inflammation and pain caused by sesamoiditis. The protocol is to use acupuncture first, then ultrasound and then ice the area for about 20 minutes. Immediately following the ice, do a deep massage of the sesamoid region, in order to break up any scar tissue or bone spurs (osteophytes) that may have developed. Do this no more than every other day for up to 4 times, every 2 weeks. This regimen is key to getting the initial inflammation to subside.

Cold laser therapy

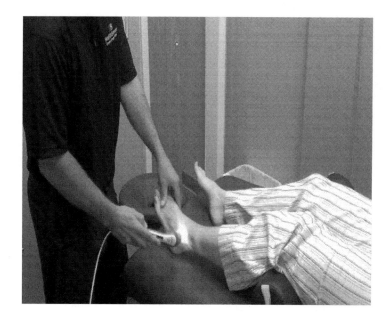

For some people cold laser therapy works better than ultrasound. If you're going to use cold laser therapy, be aware that it may require up to 10 treatments to see results, but the results can be dramatic.

Under this protocol, you'll want to do the following treatments in this order: 1) acupuncture; 2) cold laser therapy; 3) ice and then 4) deep massage of the sesamoid area to break up possible bone spurs (osteophytes).

Shockwave therapy

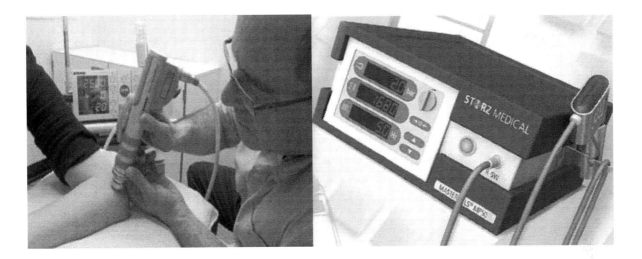

Shockwave therapy is big in Europe and is starting to come to the United States specifically for sesamoiditis. Doctors that use this type of therapy are few and far between and this form of treatment can be expensive. A Shockwave therapy session can cost up to $100 and is usually not covered by medical insurance.

Shockwave therapy worked very well for me and allowed me to run almost pain-free for up to 35 miles at a time. I used shockwave therapy every other day for two weeks. You need to stay off your foot and abstain from activity that causes inflammation in the sesamoid region while doing this therapy. I made the grave mistake of running ultras while doing this and it completely negated the effect and ended up costing me time and money.

This works very well, but it doesn't feel great. It's basically like taking a mini-hammer and pressing it up against the ball of your foot. It actually causes inflammation, but in a good way. This seems counter-intuitive, but its primary purpose is to drive blood into the area and to break up bone spurs (osteophyte).

Extracorporeal shock wave therapy (ESWT)

Extracorporeal shock wave therapy (ESWT) is a noninvasive procedure that uses sound waves to stimulate healing in some physical disorders, including tendon or tissue inflammatory disorders.

"Extracorporeal" means "outside of the body" and refers to the way the therapy is applied. Because there is no incision, ESWT offers two main advantages over traditional surgical methods: fewer potential complications and a faster return to normal activity. ESWT has been used extensively for several years to treat plantar fasciitis and other disorders.

ESWT may be considered as a therapeutic option for the patient whose sesamoid pain has not resolved with conservative treatment. Conservative measures include use of anti-inflammatory medications, steroid injections, ice packs, stretching exercises, orthotic devices (shoe inserts), and physical therapy. Some patients should not be treated with ESWT. The procedure is not appropriate for patients who have a bleeding disorder or take medications that may prolong bleeding or interfere with clotting. Your doctor or specialist will determine if the procedure is appropriate for you based on your medical history.

In preparation for ESWT, the specialist will instruct the patient to stop taking any anti-inflammatory medications (for example, aspirin or ibuprofen) for about five days before the procedure. It is important to avoid these medications because they are known to prolong bleeding under the surface of the skin.

ESWT is performed on an outpatient basis, so it does not require an overnight stay in the hospital. Before the procedure begins the patient is comfortably positioned and may receive local and/or sedation anesthesia. The treatment may take up to 30 minutes per foot. During the procedure sound waves penetrate the sesamoid area and stimulate the healing response. Sometimes more than one session is needed to adequately treat the inflammation and reduce the patient's symptoms.

The surgeon may advise you to have someone drive you home after the procedure. Other instructions may include:

• Rest and elevate the foot for the remainder of the day and night.

• Resume gentle stretching exercises the day following the procedure.

• Avoid taking any anti-inflammatory medication, such as ibuprofen or aspirin, for up to 4 weeks after ESWT.

Source: https://www.lakeviewhealth.org/upload/docs/ESWT.pdf

Over the counter orthotics

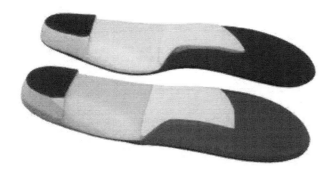

For some people, a thick over the counter orthotic like Dr. Scholls sports inserts will help correct their gait just enough to take the pressure off the forefoot and relieve pain. If you want to try an inexpensive initial solution, buy these online or at any Walgreens or CVS pharmacies. The thicker the better. I usually search on amazon.com for the best reviewed orthotics.

Custom orthotics from a sports podiatrist

Do not do this no matter what your podiatrist or orthopedic surgeon says. Custom orthotics are going to cost up to $500 per pair and are not the best product you can buy for Sesamoiditis. They're very hit or miss, and if they don't work properly, the doctor is limited in their ability to alter the orthotic because it's made by another company.

Medical insurance may or may not cover the cost of orthotics. My insurance (Blue Cross Blue Shield) covers one pair of orthotics per year.

See the section on custom orthotics made by a pedorthist.

Custom orthotics from a pedorthist

I would be willing to bet that you've never even heard the term pedorthist before. Most people haven't.

What's a pedorthist?

A pedorthist is a professional who has specialized training to modify footwear and employ supportive devices to address conditions which affect the feet and lower limbs. They're trained in the assessment of lower limb anatomy and biomechanics, and the appropriate use of corrective footwear – including shoes, shoe modifications, foot orthoses and other pedorthic devices.

A certified pedorthist assists in:

• Alleviating painful or debilitating conditions of the lower limb

• Accommodation of foot deformities

• Re-alignment of anatomical structures

• Redistribution of external and internal forces

• Improvement of balance

• Control of biomechanical function

• Accommodation of circulatory special requirements; and

• Enhancement of the actions or limbs compromised as a result of accident, congenital deformity, neural condition, or disease.

A certified pedorthist – C.Ped., or C.Ped (C) is a health professional who is trained to assess patients, formulate and implement a treatment plan and follow-up with patients. The services provided include, but are not limited to:

Assessment

The evaluation and documentation of biomechanics:

• Gait analysis including temporal and spatial assessment

• Range of motion

• Footwear analysis

• Review of potentially complicated health factors

• Circulation

• Skin integrity

• Pedorthic requirements

• Poprioception and environmental barriers including social, home and work integration.

Formulation of a treatment

• Verification of prescription/documentation.

• Evaluation of the prescription rationale.

• A needs assessment based on patient and/or caregiver input.

• Development of functional goals

• Analysis of structural and design requirements

• Consultation with and/or referral to other health care professionals as required.

Implementation of the treatment plan

• Acquisition of / modification and/or rectification of anthropometric data.

• Casting and measuring for custom footwear and/or orthotics.

• Material selection and fabrication.

• Fitting and adjusting orthoses (sometimes called orthotics).

• Fitting and modifying standard and orthopaedic footwear.

• Accommodating/incorporating complementary assistive devices.

• Fabrication of pedorthic devices.

• Device structural evaluation.

• Patient education and instruction.

Follow-up treatment plan

• Documentation of functional changes

• Formulation of modifications to ensure successful outcomes

• Reassessment of patient expectations

• Reassessment of treatment objectives

• Development of long term treatment plan

• Confirmation of patient education and instruction

This is the person you need to see in order to have custom orthotics made to address sesamoiditis. I can't stress enough how important it is to find a good pedorthist in your area. It's fairly easy to find one either online or in your local yellow pages.

A Pedorthist will know exactly how to create your orthotic in order to address your specific sesamoiditis issue. If for any reason the orthotic needs adjustment, the Pedorthist can take care of this quickly and in his office. The orthodic made by a pedorthist is almost always cheaper than the cost of the orthotic you'll get from a doctor. A Pedorthist usually makes the orthotic on-site. They'll cast your foot and talk to you about what the problem is in order to create the proper orthotic to address your specific issue.

This alone allowed me to go back to running marathons every single weekend, after nine months of not being able to run without pain. I had zero pain when I ran in the orthotics. I should also mention I had a pair of $400 orthotics made by a sports podiatrist who takes care of Olympic athletes. The orthotics did absolutely nothing to address the pain, and still allowed inflammation to occur in the area, which caused my healing time to be extended way longer than it needed to be. Allowing the sports podiatrist to make my orthotic was a mistake because the podiatrist had no way to alter the orthotic for my specific condition.

Rocker shoes

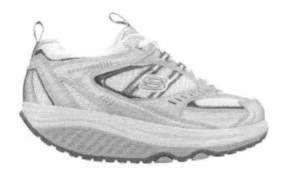

Rocker shoes will be your best friend when it comes to people who walk, hike or run often. They'll even help people who are only partially active. These shoes change your stride to take all the pressure off the forefoot. They're easy to find. If you're an ultra-runner I highly recommend rocker shoes so you never have to deal with sesamoiditis.

What if they don't make rocker shoes in my size? I have a size 15 shoe so believe me when I tell you it's difficult to find a rocker shoe in my size. The solution? See a Pedorthist. A Pedorthist or master cobbler can either create a custom rocker shoe or can take an existing shoe and modify the sole to create the rocker effect, no matter what size shoe you have.

This is a must in order to keep sesamoiditis from returning for those who got sesamoiditis just from normal walking and not from something acute.

The rocker shoes should be used in conjunction with an orthotic or dancer pad in order to alleviate any pressure on the sesamoid area. The rocker shoe does not flex much and will not allow the big toe to bend upwards which is its greatest benefit.

So who makes rocker shoes and where can you find them? Rocker shoes are pretty common these days and the best place is to search Amazon.com. Cherokee, Rockers, Avia, Skechers, Hoka, Chung Shi, among others, are brands of shoes that have a rocker model. There are all different types of rocker shoes, for all different types of problems, so make sure you do your research.

Steel shanks

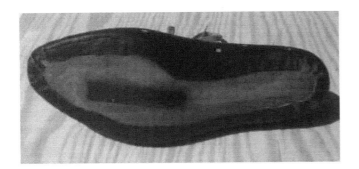

You basically have two options here: either you find a shoe with a rigid sole that doesn't flex (rocker shoe) or bend, or you have a pedorthist (or master cobbler) put a steel shank in your existing shoe to stop any sort of flex. This is something that can be done instead of wearing rocker shoes. The shank will stop the big toe from flexing or bending. One way or another, you have to make sure your big toe is not bending at all while you have any pain or inflammation.

Cortisone injections

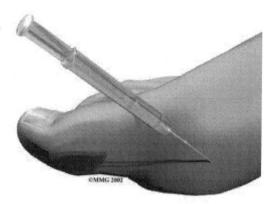

I don't recommend cortisone injections for athletes unless it's a last resort prior to a surgical solution. The reason why is that cortisone injections into the big toe joint or into the sesamoid area can lead to a rupture of the tendon as well as weakening the integrity of the area if not done correctly. Even when done correctly, there are many problems that can occur because of the cortisone. Cortisone injections do work well, but you should consult your physician to make sure this is appropriate for your particular condition. If you're fairly inactive then a cortisone injection may be appropriate, but if you follow my step by step guide to getting rid of sesamoiditis, you shouldn't need one.

NSAIDS

Nonsteroidal anti-inflammatory drugs, or NSAIDs (pronounced en-saids), are the most prescribed medications for treating conditions such as arthritis or inflammation. Most people are familiar with over-the-counter, nonprescription NSAIDs, such as aspirin and ibuprofen.

NSAIDs are more than just pain relievers. They also help reduce inflammation and lower fevers. They prevent blood from clotting, which is good in some cases but not so beneficial in others.

For example, because they reduce clotting action, some NSAIDS, especially aspirin, may have a protective effect against heart disease. However, you may bruise more easily. NSAIDs can increase the risk of developing nausea, an upset stomach, or an ulcer. They also may interfere with kidney function.

NSAIDS play a pivotal role in relieving swelling and inflammation as well as hedging against new inflammation caused by impact and use of the forefoot area. Consult your doctor before going on any sort of NSAID protocol.

There are several all-natural anti-inflammatories including substances like Tumeric that can be used if you are not able to take over the counter NSAIDS. Please consult your doctor before using any all-natural NSAID.

Topical NSAIDS or patches are another option. These provide more localized absorption directly in the area and have less impact on kidney function. Topical NSAIDS can be prescribed by your physician or sports podiatrist and ordered online or picked up at a local compound pharmacy.

Counter-irritants

Some commonly used counter-irritants contain menthol, eucalyptus oil, oil of wintergreen, camphor, eugenol from cloves, and/or turpentine oil. When rubbed on the skin, these arthritis creams or ointments create a feeling of cold or heat over the painful joint or muscle, which may help soothe painful arthritis joints. Popular brands include Therapeutic Mineral Ice, Icy Hot, and Tiger Balm.

Capsaicin

Of topical pain medications, capsaicin, an ingredient found in cayenne peppers and available in over-the-counter creams and ointments (Capzasin-P, Dolorac, Zostrix), probably has been studied the most.

Capsaicin cream warms the skin when applied over the joint and temporarily blocks a chemical called substance P, which delivers pain messages to the brain. In one study, patients with osteoarthritis or rheumatoid arthritis applied topical capsaicin four times a day to the sesamoid area. After four weeks, patients with osteoarthritis had a 33% reduction in pain; those with rheumatoid arthritis had a 57% reduction in pain. Not all studies have shown capsaicin to be this effective. Use disposable gloves when applying capsaicin cream, and avoid getting it in your eyes, nose, and mouth.

Salicylates

Other arthritis creams are available that contain salicylates, compounds related to aspirin. Using topical salicylates may help you avoid most of the side effects of taking aspirin by mouth, but how well it works to relieve pain is unclear. Some brand names include Aspercreme, Bengay, Flexall, and Sportscreme.

Lidocaine patches

Lidocaine patches are another alternative pain remedy for joint pain. Lidocaine is a drug that blocks transmission of nerve messages. It acts as an anesthetic, an agent that reduces sensation or numbs pain. In findings presented at the American Pain Society's annual meeting, researchers reported that 143 patients with osteoarthritis pain either used the Lidoderm patch, which contains lidocaine, once daily for 12 weeks or took Celebrex, an NSAID, by mouth. At 12 weeks, 71% of both groups reported at least a 30% improvement in their pain, which is considered significant pain relief.

I want to hear from you

I wrote this book to help you. I reviewed one years-worth of notes, data, meetings with doctors, blogs, websites, as well as trial and error experimenting on myself to bring you this information.

All I ask in return is that you share your stories with me and include how this book helped you. Helping people motivates me.

I know this information helped me and I know it can help you if you just follow the steps I've prescribed. Send me an email with your thoughts and stories and I'll post them on my blog and share them in future revisions to this book.

Please review my book on Amazon.com or whatever book reseller you bought from. It truly helps me out, as well as everyone else, by getting the word out to those who need this help.

About the Author

From the age of five I've been athletic and played organized sports. I think I've played just about every sport under the sun except baseball. At the age of seven, I remember going to see the movie "Chariots of Fire" with my parents. Chariots of Fire came out in 1981 so now you know how old I am. I remember being absolutely mesmerized by not only the soundtrack to the movie, but also the epic storylines of the main characters. Hell the first scene alone, when the men are running on the beach is enough to get anyone pumped up and ready to run!

From that point on, running was something ingrained in my mind. The very essence of running, the effort one has to endure and the utter feeling of gratitude one gets is something that resonates with me to my core.

When I discovered ultra-running, it was like a whole new world opened up to me. A world I had truly never known or could even have imagined. Ultra-running was the cure for everything I ever felt was wrong with my life. It makes a person a better person. And when you're the better version of yourself, you end up treating others better. I've always strived to be the best version of myself. A person who cares for others, treats others the way I'd like to be treated, and a person whose sole purpose in life is to inspire others through his own actions.

I truly believe you get what you give in life. To live a life where your prime directive is not aimed at helping others, is to live a life bereft of passion and devoid of all those things that truly matter. I used to believe that if I could choose to have any one super power, it would be the power to heal others. I've since realized that healing a physical ailment in someone can only take them so far. The true end-all-be-all super power to have is the ability to <u>inspire</u> others. No matter what anyone's problem might be, physical or emotional, the ability to inspire them is what will invoke the most powerful results.

Today, I'm an engineering systems architect. I design and implement hardware and software systems to make people's lives easier and more efficient. I'm also an endurance athlete, Ironman triathlete and ultra-distance runner. I've run over 200+ marathons, ultra-marathons and Ironman triathlons between 2012 - 2016. I will do many more.

I hate to be sidelined with injury and the engineer in me will always try and find the best solution to hedge against problems. Dealing with sesamoiditis is no different. I wrote this book to help others and to bring back hope to those who've been dealing with this problem for far too long. It's so debilitating and there just isn't any concentrated, all-encompassing help out there.

It's my greatest hope this book serves you well and that you're on your way to recovery. Thanks for reading.

To track me and my running, visit <u>www.ungermotivation.com</u>

Made in the USA
San Bernardino, CA
12 May 2018